Night Shift

10 Survival Tips for Nurses to Get Through
the Night!

Chase Hassen

Nurse Superhero

© 2015

Disclaimer:

Although the author and publisher have made every effort to ensure that the information in this book was correct at press time, the author and publisher do not assume and hereby disclaim any liability to any party for any loss, damage, or disruption caused by errors or omissions, whether such errors or omissions result from negligence, accident, or any other cause.

This book is not intended as a substitute for the medical advice of physicians. The reader should regularly consult a physician in matters relating to his/her health and particularly with respect to any symptoms that may require diagnosis or medical attention.

Contents

Introduction

Working as a nurse or nursing assistant in a hospital setting can be extremely rewarding and exciting. On every level, hospitalized patients need your help with medical care, personal care and psychosocial support.

The challenge of being a caregiver in this environment is that people are hospitalized 24 hours a day, including weekends and holidays. Shifts can be divided in half so that you work 7 am to 7 pm or 7pm to 7 am, or the more traditional 3-shift day, which generally runs as follows: 7 am to 3 pm, 3 pm to 11 pm and 11 pm to 7 am.

Regardless of the type of shift system your hospital uses, there will always be a need for nurses working during the nighttime hours, when most people are in bed sleeping. Often you may find yourself working days for a period of time, only to pick up a night shift here and there. You might also decide that working nights is more pleasurable than working days, choosing night shifts primarily and picking up some day shifts from time to time.

Our bodies thrive better on routine and the life of a hospital-based nurse is usually far from routine. In order to maintain proper physical and mental health, you need to try to make the most of the energy you have for the night shift and you need to find ways that will help you survive this kind of work.

In this book, we will look at working the night shift and hopefully fill you in on tips that can make your night job as comfortable as possible. If you can follow these tips as much as possible, you can be happy in a job that keeps you up all night

Chapter 1:
Making the Transition from Day to Night

If you have recently been hired as a full time night nurse or have decided to pick up hours for both day shifts and night shifts, you may be wondering how you can power through those nighttime hours without extreme fatigue, depression or making sleep-deprived mistakes on the job. You may also wonder if there are better ways than others to make the transition from day to nighttime shifts. These are some things you might want to do when this transition occurs:

- Recognize that working at night is not a lesson in sleep deprivation. You still need to get an average of 7-9 hours of sleep, whether it be all at once or broken up throughout the day.

- Some people simply stay awake the day before starting a night shift but this often leads to a difficult first night (or even the second or third night). You will be operating from a sleep deprived position and will be more likely to make mistakes. Sleep deprivation can bring on flu-like symptoms in which you feel sick to your stomach, exhausted and malaise.

- Consider taking a 3-4 hour nap on the evening prior to going on your first night shift. This will give you a little bit of extra energy on the first night working the late shift. Even if you can't sleep, lie down in bed and doze a little bit or watch something on television. The idea is to get the body to unwind and prepare for the burst of energy you will need to have in order to work the night shift.

- Get up and eat a light to medium-sized meal. Some people

feel better if they eat something they would ordinarily eat for breakfast, while others do fine eating a regular evening meal. Make sure you include complex carbohydrates such as whole fruits, whole vegetables, and whole grains. The importance of these foods will be discussed in the next chapter. Also include some protein, which can be in the form of dairy products, meats, beans or eggs. The combination of complex carbohydrates and protein will provide you with a steady source of energy that will last most of the night shift.

- Try to establish a routine sleep-wake cycle from the beginning. Block out the windows of your sleeping area with heavy drapes or cover the windows with tin foil while you sleep. You need to train your brain to sleep when others are not sleeping. If there will be others awake while you sleep in your home, consider buying a white noise machine to block out the footfalls and other noises that might disrupt your Earplugs can help, too. Keep a routine for the next day. You might choose to fall asleep right away after your shift or you might want to unwind and set a later time for sleeping such as from 3 pm to 10 pm or from 11 am to 6 pm for shifts starting at 7 pm. It doesn't matter what you choose to do as long as you are consistent.

- Just as you would if you worked a day shift, take a shower and dress for work. This is another habit to get into. A shower alone will help you wake up from your slumber and will help remind the body that it is time to be active and awake.

Chapter 2:
Food That Helps Us

Try not to show up to work hungry. Make sure you eat a little something containing complex carbohydrates and protein so you can increase your metabolism while you are working.

Complex carbohydrates include whole grain pasta, whole grain breads, fruits and vegetables. Starches like potatoes and sweet potatoes are complex carbohydrates as well. These are good to eat before working because they generally have a low glycemic index and will sustain your blood sugar longer than foods with high glycemic indices.

What is the glycemic index? This is an arbitrary measure of how fast the glucose sugar from your food reaches the bloodstream. Foods with a high glycemic index such as pastries, white bread, cookies and juices flood the system with glucose. While this will give you a "jolt" of energy, the insulin in the body will quickly put that sugar energy to use as part of cellular metabolism, putting the excess away as glycogen stores in your liver or as fat. When you eat foods with a high glycemic index, you can expect rapid fluctuations in your energy level and blood glucose levels. This is okay as long as you are at the peak of your glucose level but, when it inevitably crashes a few hours later, you are left with cravings for high sugar foods, junk foods and high salt foods. This yo-yo of highs and lows in your blood sugar should be avoided if at all possible.

Foods that are high in fiber will also help you regulate your blood sugars. Fiber holds onto sugar in the GI tract so that you allow the sugar to gradually be absorbed into your bloodstream. This is why foods like whole oranges are better for you than straight orange juice without the pulp. The whole orange has a lower glycemic index than the juice of the same fruit because whole oranges have more fiber in them. The same holds true for things like whole grain bread versus white bread. You regulate your blood sugars better with high fiber foods.

If you really feel shaky as though your blood sugar has reached a trough, it is okay to have something sweet to bring up your blood sugar and energy level but something like this should be the exception and not the norm.

Chapter 3:
Shifting Energy Through Meditation

Night shift work is all about shifting your energy level from being high during the day to being high at night. There are simple meditation practices that you can engage in that will help you shift your energy in the right direction.

For example, try to meditate before going to sleep. Focus on how your body feels and on the rhythmic in and out of your breathing. Relax into the meditation by relaxing your muscles in a progressive function. When you are completely relaxed, let go of the thoughts that crowd your mind, instead focusing on the here and now.

Visualization exercises can help you sleep. Imagine yourself in a beautiful place such as a beach, with its rhythmic wave motion, or imagine yourself in a forest with the rustling of leaves and the chirp of native birds. If visualization is hard for you, rent or purchase a CD or DVD that will guide you through a guided visualization pattern. It can help get you started toward being able to bring up that relaxed state of being at any time you wish.

You can also meditate before going to work or study the practice of yoga or Tai chi. These practices will energize and relax your body at the same time. You can choose to do these exercises in order to have better balance, more stamina and a relaxed state of mind. This can help you get ready for your shift or can be something you do to get rid of the stressors of the day before.

People have practiced some form of meditation and exercises like yoga, Tai chi or qi dong for many centuries, particularly in East Asian countries. Their benefits in improving energy states and calming the mind are well documented by both Eastern and

Western researches. These are activities you could work into your schedule before retiring or after you get up in preparation for your shift.

Chapter 4:
Pharmacological Agents for Nighttime Workers

If you feel you need to try and reset your biological clock, you can do this with a variety of pharmacological agents. Why might it be necessary? It's because you are naturally operating against a Circadian rhythm that marches out in the same way every day, regardless of when you work.

The Circadian rhythm involves changes in your body's hormones and other molecules that vary in amount depending on the time of day you happen to be in. For example, cortisol levels in the body vary by time of day. They tend to be higher in the morning and lower at around 10 o'clock at night. This change in cortisol level explains why children with croup or asthma tend to come into the emergency department at around this time. Their body is responding to a lower cortisol level in the evening and during the night, and there are breakthrough symptoms of wheezing and airway obstruction during this time.

When working the night shift, you are going against the natural Circadian rhythm. While there is little that can be done with regard to cortisol fluctuations throughout the day, you can definitely make an impact if you try to override the changes in melatonin levels experienced as a circadian pattern. Melatonin is a pineal gland hormone, produced by the pineal gland deep within the skull. When melatonin levels are high, you are given a bodily reminder that it is time to sleep.

Normal melatonin levels peak in the late afternoon to evening and we begin to feel sleepy. Melatonin levels drop in the morning so you feel like waking up. Fortunately, melatonin is available as a supplement. It has been found to be useful in people who have jet lag. If you take melatonin prior to sleeping during the day, you can override the natural Circadian rhythm and give the body the signal to sleep at any time during a 24 hour period of time. You still need to practice good sleep hygiene habits, including sleeping in a dark room, in a bed, and with your pajamas on. Melatonin supplementation along with good sleep habits can help you sleep when you really want to.

Benadryl ® or diphenhydramine can be used particularly when you are changing from a day job to a night job. Benadryl is an antihistamine with sedative properties. You can take 25 mg or 50 mg an hour or so before you want to sleep. It will relax you and help you drift off to sleep in a non-addicting way.

There are prescription benzodiazepines you can use to reset your sleep-wake cycle; however, they can be habit forming and are not recommended as part of an ongoing routine of getting to sleep.

Avoid caffeine or alcohol before retiring as both can contribute to insomnia. Smoking, too, before sleep can make it difficult to get to sleep. It is far better to eat a light meal and drink a cup of green tea than it is to take in anything that might keep you awake. If sleep deprivation becomes a problem and you have tried everything, seek medical attention to get you through the difficult task of changing your nights to days and vice versa.

Chapter 5:
Make Use of Your Break Time

Unless things are extraordinarily busy, you should be able to have a meal break or even a 15 minute break sometime during your shift. Some people feel comfortable eating during this time. It should be known, however, that research has shown that people who work night shifts tend to choose foods to eat that aren't particularly healthy for you. Pack a healthy lunch and stick to eating what you have brought with you instead of the candy in the vending machine or the doughnuts a coworker brought.

If you can eat on the job, spread the meal over the course of several hours rather than eating everything at once. Try going to a break room and take a short nap instead. Rather than making you even more tired, a short 15-20 minute nap can revive you for the rest of your shift. Be sure someone awakens you after your nap or set an alarm. It is too easy to slip into a nighttime sleeping pattern if you sleep longer than 30 minutes at a stretch during your shift. Take turns with other likeminded nurses so you can cover each other's patients while you nap during your break time.

You can also choose your break time to become a time for a quick walk around the hospital. The change in scenery and the muscle activity will get your heart rate going and you can begin to build up the energy that is lost when you have to sit behind a nursing desk all night long.

Engage others in conversation if more than one of you is breaking at the same time. A relaxing conversation with a coworker can strengthen the bond you will ultimately have with coworkers who are struggling with being night staff at the hospital. It is too easy to focus more on how hard it is to work the night shift and less on building the camaraderie necessary for a successful work life.

Remember that you are not in this alone and others are trying to cope with having a topsy turvy work life in the same way you are.

Chapter 6:
Handling Stress

Some people prefer working nights because the pace is slower and the patients are, for the most part, bedded down for the night. If your work load permits, spend some time reading charts or even reading a few pages from a novel during the slow periods.

As previously mentioned, the bond between night workers tends to be greater than the bond between day workers. You should have more time to get to know the lives of your coworkers when working at night. This camaraderie can bring on more energy and interest in your night job. Getting to know your coworkers is perhaps the best step you can make in reducing the stress of working nights and in finding a sounding board for the stressors you experience away from work. Think of your nocturnal coworkers and you belonging to a special club of people performing a valuable duty while the rest of the world sleeps. You need these people to get you through your shift and it is likely they need you as well.

You are in a uniquely stressful situation when you work the night shift. In general, patients sleep and the general tone of the nighttime is one of restfulness. The hallway lights may even be dimmer at night, contributing to sleepiness on the job. But then again, anything can happen unexpectedly during the night shift and you may have to go from having a slow evening to having someone crash in the middle of the night, bringing in more staff and doctors to deal with the crisis. This pattern of little stress punctuated by high periods of stress can be very difficult to tolerate and can add to your personal feelings of stress around your job.

These are the same things doctors, firefighters and ambulance personnel must deal with in the course of their night shifts. It means that, even when things are quiet, just about anything can happen at any time. Prepare your mind and body for this inevitability by relaxing when you can so you can be prepared for when all hell breaks loose.

It takes a special person to work the night shift. Some people find themselves getting biochemically depressed if they work the night shift for a long period of time. You can't really know if you are the type of person who can withstand the rigors of night time wakefulness and daytime slumber unless you give it a try. If you have a personal or family history of depression, take special note that you might develop symptoms of depression even though you like your job and the people you are working with. Some of it may be genetic and something you can overcome only by switching to a day job or by trying to make do with an antidepressant that can change your natural biochemical response to the stress of a night job.

Chapter 7:
Time Management

During the night shift, there are commonly fewer people to do the same work that more people shared during the day shift. Patients still need observation, pain medications, bathroom trips and bed pans. Rarely is the night shift a completely quiet job—like babysitting for a sleeping baby. Patients need attention and you may have up to twice as many patients to carry out your work as do day nurses.

Some of this added stress on your time management skills is warranted. There are fewer people visiting the sick, fewer procedures scheduled, fewer surgeries and a quieter telephone. Patients are rarely discharge in the middle of the night although admissions can come on any shift.

With fewer people on the ward to do the work of nurses, aides, and station coordinators, you'll need to manage your time a bit better than you would during the day. For example, you might have a patient that needs the assistance of two in order to use the bathroom in the middle of the night and the number of aides to help is usually less than during the day. This means that RNs and other staff need to work together to accomplish things—sharing the workload so you aren't stuck doing something that would be better managed with two persons.

The night time shift is not the time to be selfish or refuse to help your coworker when they need help with their patient. You may need the same help from the same coworker in a few hours and it pays off to help others so you can get help in return. From a time management perspective, it makes sense. You can collaborate on a difficult task with a coworker in less time than it would take you to do the same job by yourself. Extend that same favor to a coworker when they need your help and tasks get accomplished much faster and with greater efficiency.

While you may have an assigned number of patients, the truth of the matter is that time management for the night shift means you will have to take part in the care of another nurse's patients, either during his or her break or when the load requires two people to accomplish the task. In a sense, you are time managing for the whole team of nurses and other staff who are operating at night. The more you collaborate with others on the night shift, the faster things will get done and the less stress you will feel.

Just as in the day shift, you will have to chart your progress as the night goes on. Try not to save it until the early morning hours because anything could happen when you have set aside a time for charting and you will find yourself unprepared to give report to the day shift. Because the nighttime shift involves periods of quite punctuated by periods of chaos (more so than is seen during the daytime shift), you should take the quiet opportunities to update your progress. That way, regardless of what happens at the end of your shift, you will be well on your way toward finishing your charting without the stress of being unprepared.

Night time isn't just about watching over sleeping patients. You may have to prepare a patient for surgery; you may have to struggle with nighttime pain management with one of your patients; you might have a patient that is on the nurse's button all night long because they have to use the restroom or are scared and anxious at night. You need to think about these possibilities during every shift so you can have the paperwork and other necessities of charting done when things are slower. The goal is to be as "done" as possible when the next shift arrives. The better you have managed your time, the sooner will you be able to give a complete report on the patients you are caring for. This means getting off duty at a reasonable hour so you can go home to sleep or to see your kids off to school.

Chapter 8:
Exercise for Night Time Work

One big problem night shift workers face is the natural gravitation toward eating junk food in order to stay awake. People bring in treats or use the vending machine in order to get something that will give them that quick burst of energy they need to fight off fatigue. In general, this means that night shift workers are at a greater risk for being overweight or obese when compared to daytime workers.

One way to manage this is through diet and exercise. We've talked about diet and the need to even out the blood sugar energy throughout the day and night. But what about the role of exercise in reducing the chance of becoming obese and the inherent health risks that go with it—things like diabetes, certain cancers and heart disease? Obesity can tip the scales of health toward a situation of poor health and a shortened lifespan.

Unless you do a lot of physical exercise on the job, it means you need to exercise at some point in the day. When is the right time to exercise and what kinds of exercises are appropriate for a night shift worker?

The best way to manage exercise in night shift workers is to engage in approximately 30 minutes of aerobic exercise on most, if not all, the days of the week. Aerobic exercise is the type of exercise you do that raises your heart rate, your respiratory rate and gets your body moving. This is opposed to anaerobic exercise such as Pilates and weight lifting. When you work out on weight machines at the gym, this is also anaerobic exercise.

A good way to plan an exercise program is to do about 5 sessions of aerobic exercise in any given week, with anaerobic activity the other two days of the week. While anaerobic exercise like weight lifting doesn't burn as many calories as anaerobic exercise, it does increase muscle mass. The more muscle you have, the greater will be your metabolic rate. In other words, people who have a greater muscle mass will burn more calories at rest than will a person with less muscle mass.

Anaerobic exercise, particularly those weight lifting activities that strengthen your core muscles, will be helpful to you in your job as well. You will have less back pain and will be able to move patients from gurney to bed or from one spot in their bed to the other without undue stress on your back. Back injuries are all too common in nursing because of the lifting that must be done on a nightly basis when turning patients or helping them get out of bed to use the restroom or commode.

Pilates makes for a good exercise for nurses because it strengthens the core muscles of the back and abdomen so you will strain yourself less when using these muscles at work. Exercise machines that are targeted toward improving abdominal muscles and back muscles are also good exercises to consider as preparation for the clinical care of the hospitalized patient.

Aerobic activity should be done approximately 5 times per week for about thirty minutes at a stretch. Aerobic exercise can be anything from walking, jogging, cycling, swimming, golf, tennis, or any other activity that gets you moving.

When should you do this kind of activity if you are a night shift worker? It all depends on when you choose to sleep. If you stay up until later in the afternoon to sleep, you should exercise shortly after coming home from work. Any activity you do should be about 4-5 hours before retiring. This is because exercise increases your metabolic rate and can activate you to the point of having difficulty falling asleep. Even though it makes you tired after exercise, there is the "runner's high" factor to consider and the fact that exercise right before sleep is known to decrease your ability to drift off to sleep.

If you go to bed right away after you get off from the night shift, you can do your exercise just after getting up in the afternoon. This will increase your metabolic rate throughout the afternoon and evening, even several hours after the exercise is over. By the time you are off to work, the effects of the exercise will largely have worn off with the exception of the fact that you will have burned more calories during the day and will have a better chance of avoiding becoming overweight.

There are advantages of trying the ancient arts of qi dong, Tai chi and yoga. All will increase your flexibility and strength but they do so in a way that nourishes the mind as well. In Tai chi, you engage in fluid-like movements done along with breathing exercises and mindfulness. There is deep meditation in doing Tai chi that can calm your mind throughout your day. The same can be said for qi dong, another Chinese-based exercise. Qi dong also involves movements, meditation and muscle strengthening but it is a milder form of exercise than Tai chi and can be done by anyone at just about any fitness level.

Yoga combines muscle flexibility through various poses, breathing exercises and meditation. There are several different types of yoga to choose from, including "hot yoga", which is done in a very hot room. Hatha yoga is a common form of yoga practiced at health clubs all over America. It is gentler than hot yoga and can be done without any particular equipment or a significant history of exercising.

These ancient forms of exercise are particularly good for night shift workers in that they foster a tight mind-body connection and can relieve some of the stressors of the job. You can purchase a DVD to teach you these types of exercises. Health clubs are increasingly offering classes in the Eastern exercise programs and, if you choose that route, there are more opportunities for you to socialize and stay in contact with the waking world.

Chapter 9:
Take Care of Yourself

It is easy to feel left out of the world's activities when you work nights and sleep during the day. While you are sleeping, your loved ones are going about their own business and you are often not included because it would interfere with your much needed sleep. The trick to successfully becoming a night shift worker is to take care of your mind and body and to maintain contact with the waking world as much as you can.

How can you take care of yourself better as a night shift worker? Here are some thoughts:

- Keep a set sleep-wake cycle. While it is tempting to go without a full day's sleep in order to be with family or get your chores done, you need to reset your sleep-wake cycle in such a way that you go to bed at the same time and get up at the same time. Just when you choose to make your sleep time depends on what works for you. Some people adopt a pattern of having two separate but long sleep episodes with time in the middle of the day to shop, exercise, clean your house or be with family. If this works for you and adds up to a 7-9 hour period of quality sleep, then try it. The faster you can get a routine going of sleeping and being awake at the same time in a 24 hour period of time, the better you will function in your waking hours, including the hour spent at work.

  When it is your day off, it is tempting to revert to a nighttime sleeping habit just for those days. The problem is that this simply confuses your body and mind; you will have a tougher time getting back to a routine work schedule if you blow the whole sleep-wake cycle out of the water on your days off. Stick to your sleeping schedule even if it is your day off and you will be doing your body a favor.

- Stay away from highly processed foods and foods high in sugar and salt. These are often empty calories that do not add up to a good nutritional state. Take the time to cook healthy foods using fruits, vegetables, lean meats, beans and complex carbohydrates in the form of high fiber whole grains. Your gastrointestinal tract has its own rhythm that can get seriously thrown off if you don't keep a set schedule. Constipation and/or diarrhea are common phenomena of night shift workers because they attempt to eat and sleep at times not conducive to having regular bowel movements. As you continue to eat healthy foods at regular intervals throughout the day, your GI tract will respond to this change over time and you will develop a different yet perfectly acceptable time for regular bowel movements at whatever time of day your body settles into your new schedule.

- Treat yourself to a massage every so often—at least once per month. You are doing hard work throughout the night and, especially if you are under stress, you need the nimble fingers and hands of a good massage therapist to get the kinks out of stressed out muscles. Massage therapy can be done at any time of the day but it is especially helpful if done right before retiring for the day. Take a warm shower if the oil on your skin after a massage bothers you but you can otherwise drift off to sleep with the fragrance of your massage oil on your body.

- Keep up with what's going on in your life while you've been sleeping. Find time to be with family that works with your new sleep-wake cycle so you can keep up with their day and with the events going on around the world while you were sleeping. This will help you feel less like a mole or other nocturnal animal and more like a human being. Elicit the help from your loved ones by asking them to respect your new sleep-wake cycle by being as quiet as they can be while you sleep. There are enough difficulties in sleeping during the day that are only made worse by excess noise coming from other parts of the house.

- As mentioned, consider buying a white noise machine or one that plays the sounds of the ocean or other nature sounds. When you do this, you are sending the mind the signal it needs to let you know you are going to sleep. It blocks out unwanted noise and will help you sleep better. Some people keep the white noise machine going all night long while others use it on a timer system to naturally shut off after about 90 minutes. Experiment to see what works best for you.

- Fight off obesity through healthy eating and exercise. Exercise is especially important in night shift workers because it allows for time to raise your metabolic rate so you can shed excess pounds and will be more likely to refuse the doughnuts or other treats people bring to help pass the time during the night shift. If you don't have the time to exercise during the day, try walking during your break time at work. Hospitals are filled with corridors for walking and you can take the stairs from one floor to the next as part of your exercise program. Exercise fights off mental fatigue, which is a common problem in night shift workers—even more than physical fatigue. Do your best to burn off excess calories by having an exercise routine that fits your new sleep-wake pattern.

Chapter 10:
Keep Your Social Contacts Alive

Perhaps one of the more difficult things to tolerate when you become a night shift worker is that you are sleeping when many of your old friends are awake and engaging in activities you would rather be doing than sleeping. Keep in telephone contact as much as possible with friends and loved ones. You might have to adjust your sleep-wake cycle on occasion in order to be able to go out to dinner, enjoy a show or even play cards with people who will be drifting off to sleep just as your work day begins. There is usually some overlap time in which both you and your loved ones are naturally awake. Make use of those times to their fullest. Nothing is more depressing than not being able to spend time with loved ones and friends who are sleeping while you are awake or who are awake while you really need your sleep. Just because you work nights doesn't make you a freak or an outcast in your social circle. It only means that you have to make an extra effort to be included in activities and leisure time along with your friends.

You may find it easier to do things with other people who have the same sleep-wakeful schedule as you do. For example, befriend a coworker who works your same shift and who wouldn't mind going to a matinee movie with you before you both go home to sleep before the next shift. Think of it as an opportunity to expand your social sphere rather than a time to hole up in your bedroom sleeping all day. Night shift work at the hospital often offers enough down time so you can share your life and your history with people who like being social at work. There is a common bond you share with other night shift workers and this can continue to grow outside of the workplace at times when both you and your coworkers are awake.

Try to instill on your day shift friends the idea that you need time to sleep uninterrupted by phone calls from them during the time you are sleeping. If they don't respect your wishes to the fullest, try having the phone be as far from your sleep time as possible. Let someone else in your family pick up the phone and take a message from you. If you get a lot of annoying sales calls throughout the day and if there is no one to field these calls, put your phone on silent mode and use an answering machine to take messages for you. It is tough enough to sleep during the day without having to take phone calls from solicitors or even from your friends and loved ones. It is a matter of remembering your priorities and setting limits on those people who try to violate your boundaries around sleeping and being awake.

Conclusion

Whether the night shift is your chosen passion or is just the only job you can get at this time, you can turn it into a positive experience that you will learn and grow from. Because night shift work goes against your body's natural Circadian rhythm, you will experience an adjustment period at first where you feel an inordinate tendency to want to sleep at night and be awake in the daytime like everyone else. Some of the adjustment is purely biological and depends on fluctuations in hormones that are not conducive to night shift work.

Night shift work requires attention to your emotional health as well. If you are prone to depression or bipolar disorder, working the night shift can precipitate symptoms. As mentioned, see your doctor if you feel as though you are becoming depressed or anxious because of your work schedule. Medications are available that can help the biological component of major depression and bipolar disorder.

Driving your motor vehicle in the first week or so after starting night shift work may take special attention on your part because your mind will not have adjusted to the change in your sleep-wake cycle, leaving you sleep deprived and more prone to accidents and mistakes on the road. Know that this will pass after a few weeks and that you will be able to drive to work and back to home without nodding off at the wheel.

Try melatonin if you want a quicker fix to your sleeping woes. It is a completely safe and natural hormone that can be used for long periods of time without an addictive potential. If melatonin does not help you reset your sleep-wake cycle, talk to your doctor about getting a mild sleep-inducing medication that you will use for just a few weeks until your body adjusts naturally to your new schedule. Some people may be prescribed tricyclic antidepressant medication such as amitriptyline or nortriptyline, which are naturally sedating, not addictive and can fight off night shift depression. You can take tricyclic antidepressants to adjust your sleep schedule and you can safely use it for long periods of time without risk of dependency.

Take care of your body through proper diet and exercise. Researchers have found a link between night shift working or rotating schedules and an increased risk of heart disease, obesity, diabetes and stomach trouble, such as stomach ulcers. Rather than sit back and let these diseases come to you, take the initiative to eat for lower cholesterol levels, a normal weight and a diet rich in antioxidants which scavenge for oxygen free radicals implicated in cellular damage and cancer.

While you can't be sure that doing the night shift is something you want to do as a regular job, especially in the beginning, try to go easy on your body during this time to give yourself the best chance of success at work. Eat foods that come from your kitchen and not from a fast food take out place or from a vending machine. Sleep and awaken at the same time every day and keep your social life as alive as possible while you are working nights. The feelings of isolation alone can contribute to health problems caused by excess stress, worry and anxiety.

Your true friends will understand your need to sleep during the day for a proper number of hours and will avoid calling you or forcing you to go out on the town during the times when you should be sleeping.

Avoid the pitfalls of caffeine, alcohol and nicotine if you choose to be a night worker. If you have become used to drinking coffee in the morning to wake up, you can continue this habit when you awaken before going to your night shift. Just don't take caffeine pills and sedative medications to force your body into a state that is unnatural and harmful to your health. Night shift workers are running against the grain of what society and our biological clocks are telling us. This is the time to take care of your body by avoiding unnatural chemicals that only mimic a normal sleep-wake cycle.

Allow yourself time to adjust to the new routine. Be especially careful about your sleep habits and listen to your body if it is telling you that you are becoming sleep deprived. Anything less than 7 hours of sleep at a stretch will set you up for sleep deprivation and all the dangers this condition causes. You will make fewer mistakes at work and will be a better driver if you start in the beginning by taking care of your body through sleep, exercise and healthy eating.

You don't have to suffer through working the night shift. If it is not for you, feel free to find another job that allows you to sleep at night. But, if you are one of the 8.6 million Americans who choose to do shift work or just work the night shift, know that there will be an adjustment period before your body adjusts to the change in sleeping patterns. Because you have a higher risk of stroke, metabolic syndrome, heart attacks, infertility, diabetes, and obesity just by choosing to work at night, you will have to set the tone toward better health habits from the beginning so you can counteract these health risks.

It is possible to live a full and healthy life as a night shift worker if you are careful to listen to your mind and body and if you adopt healthy lifestyle habits early on in your career. Don't forget to be social to whatever degree you can be and set boundaries about sleep and wakefulness that will keep you from a bad cycle of sleep deprivation and poor work performance that can happen if you don't take care of yourself.

I want to thank you for purchasing my book! I hope you really enjoyed it. If so, do you mind doing me a quick favor and writing a review on amazon? Reviews are very important and help me to connect with more people just like you!

I'll talk to you soon and see you in the next book!

- Chase Hassen

Nurse Superhero

www.ingramcontent.com/pod-product-compliance
Lightning Source LLC
Chambersburg PA
CBHW070757180526
45168CB00004B/1644